TABLE OF CONTENTS

I0427846

How To Fix Thinning Hair Manual

A Step By Step Guide For Growing Thicker Hair

AUTHOR BREANNA RUTTER

INTRODUCTION TO
THE THINNING HAIR MANUAL

"The How To Fix Thinning Hair Manual is a pocket guide that will help you to successfully revert your thinning hair to achieve thicker hair! There are a variety of reasons that could have caused your hair to thin such as; health issues, aggressive styling, or a natural progression of thinning from aging. Growing back thicker hair is possible and your process to doing so will include a wide array of solutions that range from topical thickening treatments, hairstyling and maintenance habits and even the option to go the surgical route if you so choose! Understanding how to revert thinning hair can be quite challenging especially when patience comes into play because it is required to wait a period of time in conjunction with the natural growth cycle of your hair to allow yourself time to recover and see results.

This manual breaks down growing back thicker hair in simple easy steps involving growth treatments, hair care regimens and the option of dieting for thickness and so much more! The skills required to achieve thicker hair are of a minimum skill level paired with a vast array of hair knowledge so that you can understand why you have to do certain things to your hair, to maintain and encourage the health of it. This manual is here to thoroughly educate you about your hair as well as provide a multitude of solutions that will help you to grow your hair thick and healthy.

Please enjoy this informative read and remain patient throughout the process as you are growing thicker hair!"

Sincerely Breanna

1 HAIR GROWTH CYCLE

Understanding the life cycle of hair will give you the basic foundation of knowing how to diagnose a variety of problems you may encounter when recovering from thinning hair. Knowing the behavioral characteristics of hair growth will indicate whether or not your hair is growing properly, if the shedding you may experience is normal and also how quickly you can expect to see thicker growth results. Knowing how long you should expect your hair to revert from thinning is crucial towards knowing if your growing efforts are really making difference!

Hair encounters three stages within its growth or life cycle. Each individual hair you are growing on your head can be in different stages of its life cycle and because of that, you lose on average 80 to 100 strands of hair daily. Given that you have about 100,000 strands of hair on your head in total, don't be alarmed about shedding that many strands because this is a normal process that has to takes place. If you think about it, shedding makes up way less than 1% of hair that you have on your scalp right now! Now let's discuss the life cycle of hair.

The Anagen Phase is the 1st phase of the hair life cycle as this is the growing phase because a new hair has begun growing. Since all of your hair is not in the Anagen Phase at once, it will take time before you will notice thickness because other hairs have to enter this phase as well. This phase lasts 2 to 6 years.

The Catagen Phase is the 2nd phase in which your hair is transitioning towards the Telogen phase. The hair is separating from your follicle (see definition guide) and moving upward towards your pore, or the surface of your scalp to fall out as shed hair. This phase lasts 1 to 2 weeks.

The Telogen Phase is the 3rd phase in which the hair is resting because the dermal papilla (see definition guide) separates from the follicle and then moves upward to begin growing a brand new hair. This phase lasts 2 to 4 months.

It is important that you completely understand the hair growth cycle so that you can gauge how long it should take for your thinning hair to begin showing signs of improvement! The Telogen Phase and the Anagen Phase are the only two phases that allows you to see growth in hair. The time frames between the two phases are 2 months to 6 years. You should not have to wait 6 years to see your hair thicken because remember, all hair is not in the same phase at the same time!

The golden time frame to stick with when trying to reverse thinning hair is no longer than 2 to 4 months time to notice changes. You should see your hair begin to thicken in as little as 2 months and if you do not see results, 4 months is the longest time you need to wait to see changes with your hair.

If you remain consistent in trying a specific recommendation as instructed for thickening thinning hair, and you see no signs of change within 2 to 4 months, go ahead and try another recommendation until you find success with reversing your thin hair!

2 UNDERSTANDING HAIR PH

Have you ever experienced difficulty maintaining smooth or tame hair? Frizzy hair will ruin any hairstyle and unruly hair seems to show most when straightened or in braids and twists. The reason why frizzy or unruly hair is hard to tame is because the hair is not PH balanced! PH balance has a lot to do with the health and behavior of your hair to achieve certain results. In relation to thinning hair, hair is left prone to breakage and further thinning if your hair is not maintained its ideal range of PH!

The PH scale is used to measure how acidic or alkaline a solution is and the scale ranges from 1 (acidic) to 14 (alkaline). Water has a PH of 7 (neutral) and is used to compare the acidity or alkalinity of a solution. The ideal PH range of hair is 4.5 to 5.5. Hair has an acidity of 4.5 to 5.5 and should remain this way especially if you want to achieve your most healthy hair. The reason why this is important is because when your hair is in contact with an acidic product, it will cause your cuticles (refer to definition guide) to flatten resulting in smooth & healthy moisturized strands of hair. When hair is in contact with an alkaline solution, the cuticles raise, the strands themselves swell (which can cause breakage) resulting in rough, unruly and frizzy dry hair.

When caring for your hair, it is high priority to maintain a PH range of 4.5 to 5.5 and a great way to do this, is to make sure that your hair care products are PH balanced. If you do not know the PH of your hair care products, test your products with Litmus Strips. You can find these strips in specialty stores and online. If you want products that are already PH balanced, I highly suggest HowToBlackHair.com referred hair care products specifically formulated for maintaining healthy hair.

3 THICKENING HAIR GROWTH OILS

There are a multitude of hair care products available on the market that offer to repair a variety of hair problems many individuals suffer from today. Visit a local drug store to check out the beauty isle to inspect the hair care products. You will notice that most of the hair care products offer repair for problems such as split ends, fading color, flat thin hair and so on! The problem is that many products that promise to thicken hair are not actually formulated with ingredients that contribute to those effects! When reading the labels of many commercialized hair care products, you will notice that the most popular products are filled with ingredients such as; petrolatum, silicones, and sulfates! These are the worst ingredients known for hair because they cause buildup, breakage, and dry hair! To grow back thicker hair, it is best to make sure that you are using ingredients that strengthen your hair from the inside out, encourage blood flow for optimal hair growth, and keep your hair PH balanced.

On the following pages are recipes for thickening your hair and a regimen that you can use and follow along with in the comfort of your own home to help you to reverse your thin or thinning hair. Please keep in mind the growth cycle of hair is in between 2 months to 6 years so give yourself 2 to 4 months, courtesy of the Anagen Phase, to truly see results with your hair. If one recipe does not improve your hair as suggested, move onto another treatment after 4 months to find the solution that works best for you!

Always perform a 24 hour patch test in a discrete area of your head. All recipes contribute to thicker hair & some recipes simultaneously offer the benefit of treating other hair issues as well!

OIL RECIPES FOR THICKENING HAIR

(Recipes are created based on how well the scents complement one another)(For the highest nutritional quality of oil, choose Unrefined Cold Pressed Virgin Oils)

Lavender Oil Blend
(For Thickness)

6 drops of Lavender Essential Oil
1 tbsp. of Castor Oil
1 tbsp. of Coconut Oil

Ylang Ylang Oil Blend
(Thickness + Strength)

6 drops of Ylang Ylang Essential Oil
1 ounce (2 tbsp.) of Grass Fed Butter Oil

Jamaican Black Castor Oil
(Thickness + Strength)

1 ounce (2 tbsp.) of Jamaican Black Castor Oil

Bay Oil Blend
(For Stronger Hair)

6 drops of Bay Essential Oil
1 tbsp. of Argan Oil
1 tbsp. of Avocado Oil

THICKENING OIL APPLICATION + REGIMEN

THIS CAN BE DONE DAILY!

Step #1 Use an applicator bottle to apply thin lines of Thickening Hair Oil Recipe onto your scalp.

Step #2 Message scalp with the pads of your fingers for about 5 minutes to increase blood flow and allow oil to penetrate your scalp.

Step #3 Rub oily hands down hair to treat your remaining hair.

For straighter hair, use a paddle brush to help distribute oils throughout your hair. For course or kinky hair, it is preferred to use your hands to prevent breakage from constant combing or brushing while distributing oils.

4 DETANGLE REGIMEN

The Detangling Regimen for thin hair is a vital technique that must be done appropriately every single time you need to detangle your hair! Detangling your hair should never be performed often and improperly for a couple of reasons; excessive detangling causes breakage and constant detangling overtime will lead to excessive thinning. The most difficult part about detangling has always been encountering knots and tangles and even more daunting than that, grooming course or thin hair!

Thin Hair: your ponytail width, with all of your hair gathered, is the width of a nickel or smaller

Course Hair: your individual strands of hair are the same size or bigger in size (diameter) to regular sewing thread

Even if you do not have thin and/or course hair, that does not mean detangling is any easier than someone with thicker hair considering that fact when thin course hair encounters hair damage, the damage is pronounced and even more difficult to conceal!

Provided next is a detangling regimen for thin or thinning hair to ensure that you will not suffer from furthermore damage as you are trying to thicken your hair. For more information on specific detangling regimens, check out The Transitioning Hair Manual, The Relaxed Hair Bible, or The Natural Hair Bible if you need detailed hair care instructions and hair care regimens for growing longer and healthier hair.

DETANGLE REGIMEN
FOR THIN OR THINNING HAIR

Step #1 Moisten hair with a water spray bottle and wait a couple of minutes for hair to soften.

Step #2 GENTLY separate hair into manageable sections (about 6 to 8 sections of hair).

Step #2 For course hair, apply a rinse conditioner to hair before detangling with a seamless wide tooth comb and for fine hair, treat hair with your Thickening Oil Recipe of choice before detangling.

Step #3 For course hair, rinse out conditioner with warm water, pat towel dry and treat hair with Thickening Oil Recipe of choice.

Step #4 After applying your Thickening Oil Recipe of choice, two strand twist to allow hair to air dry or proceed to style according to taste.

DO NOT APPLY ANY ADDITIONAL PRODUCT TO YOUR HAIR WHATSOEVER !

5 NIGHT TIME ROUTINE

Your night time routine is vital for preserving the health of your hair and without this routine, you will constantly suffer from breakage and thinning hair. Not only does handling your hair in a gentle manner dramatically decrease breakage and thinning, but so does your protective night time routine!

When performing your night time routine, it is very important that your hair has been already prepped with your Thickening Hair Oil Application. Before going to bed, you must always protect with appropriate material. The two choices of fabric that are best for protecting your hair throughout the night are Satin and Silk.

Satin is more affordable than silk, more flexible material than silk, and can be washed with ease. Satin does not cause friction on your hair and nor does Silk, but Satin will cause more friction in comparison to Silk.

Silk is priced higher than satin, is not as flexible in comparison satin, and has to be delicately hand washed or cleansed through a dry cleaning service. Silk does not cause friction on your hair and nor does Satin, but Silk is superior in preventing friction than Satin.

There are a few ways to protect your hair from friction with Silk or Satin material such as using a; Satin/Silk Pillowcase, Bonnet or Head Scarf. For preserving healthy hair, it is preferred to sleep with a Bonnet or Scarf to keep the hair neat with no movement throughout the night.

Follow the suggested night time routine to protect your hair to eliminate friction and breakage.

NIGHT TIME ROUTINE

Step #1 Perform The Thickening Hair Oil Application

Step #2 (For Satin/Silk Pillowcase)

Cover your bed pillow of choice with your case of choice. Double case your pillow if needed because of slippage.

Step #3 (For Satin/Silk Bonnet)

Wear a comfortable but secure bonnet that covers all of your hair including your edges. If the bonnet feels tight or too loose to stay secure, seek another bonnet or protection of choice.

Step #4 (For Satin/Silk Head Scarf)

Secure your scarf around your head in a way that covers all of your hair including your edges.

IMPORTANT Alternate the tied knot of your head scarf in a new position on your hairline every night. Constantly knotting the scarf at the same point along your hairline will lead to more thinning!

6 HAIRSTYLING OPTIONS

You must carefully consider your choice of hair styling options especially in regards to using extensions to require a certain look while also preserving the health of your hair. Often times, hairstyling is the culprit to many who suffer from thinning hair! Below are lists of some of the worst and best hairstyles to wear to while trying to thicken your thin hair. One important thing to remember is that the more hairs contained within a given braid or twist, the stronger your hair will be in numbers.

WORST HAIRSTYLES TO WEAR WITH THIN HAIR
Micro Braids – small braids cause thinning easily
Kinky Twist (small) – small twists cause thinning easily
Ponytail Sew In – exposed hair edges/nape can thin easily
Partial Sew In – leave out experiences thinning easily
Yarn Braids – yarn is too heavy for thin hair
Yarn Wraps – yarn is too heavy for thin hair
U-Part/L-Part Wig – leave out experiences thinning easily
Quick Weave – thin hair will tear from glue removal

BEST HAIRSTYLES TO WEAR WITH THIN HAIR
Jumbo Individual Braids – large braids decrease breakage
Kinky Twists (large) – large twists decrease breakage
Net Weave Full Sew In – tension is on net instead of hair
Invisible Part Sew In – all thin hair is concealed

Even though there are more choices than listed here for best hairstyles, it is most important to not add additional products, weaves or extensions to thin hair to ultimately avoid setbacks while thickening your hair. Opt to slick down your hair while damp with a molding strip instead of applying tension from styles. It will not hold as well as using hair gel but you can use hair gel once you reverse your thinning hair.

7 HEAT USAGE

Using heat on thin hair is dangerous towards preserving the health of your hairs while trying to thicken them! Heat should only be used rarely even on healthy hair so when it comes to attaining thicker hair, using heat is never appropriate for the most part. The only time heat usage is appropriate is if you are doing a Deep Conditioning or Protein Treatment. In this case, heat is used all over you hair to encourage your products to penetrate your hair. If the heat is only focused on the edges of your hair for example, this will cause your hair to become weakened which results in more thinning and breakage.

Some individuals think that if you use heat regularly with a heat protectant it will prevent any cause of breakage when this is totally false! First, before you even bring yourself to using a heat straightener or heat styling tool on your hair, you have to test which setting is best for you. Your preferred heat setting of choice should be the lowest setting on your styling tool that allows you to achieve your straightest result. For some, especially with fine or thin hair, their heat setting usually falls somewhere between 300° and 320° degrees. For those usually with thick or coarse hair, their heat setting will usually fall between 320° to 350°

On healthy hair, moderating your frequency of heat usage, along with using a heat protectant product at your lowest straightening heat setting that works for you, should protect your hair from heat damage. The only way the above suggestion will damage your hair is if your hair is unhealthy! Unhealthy hair is on the brink of breakage and that is why you have to make sure that your thin or thinning hair becomes healthy first, to avoid sacrificing any progress you are trying to make in regards achieving thicker healthy hair!

8 CHEMICAL RELAXERS

Some of those who are reading this manual may have relaxed hair, and relaxing your hair should not ruin your thin hair if done appropriately. Always use chemical relaxers with caution and stretch your touch ups as far apart from one another as possible because breakage and thinning is always a risk when chemically relaxing your hair!

Chemical relaxers and their dangers are heavily discussed in my book, The Relaxed Hair Bible: The 10 Commandments of Long Healthy Relaxed Hair so if you want to learn concentrated information on their usage, regimens, hair care treatments and more, refer to that books for detailed information. It's very important to understand the dangers of using chemical relaxers when trying to grow thicker hair. Since this manual is focused on growing thicker hair and doing everything possible to also keep your hair healthy, it is suggested to stop chemically relaxing your hair!

This may be hard advice to follow for those who chose to chemically relax their hair but if you do chose to postpone your touch ups until you have attained thicker hair, this will guarantee you the most success with progressing with your hair. As discussed in the Relaxed Hair Bible, chemical relaxers are highly alkaline and by nature, they disintegrate (or break down) your hairs to the point of straightness. When a relaxer is left on for too long or too high of strength is used, this can cause your hair to melt or simply break off and become thin. As mentioned in chapter two titled, Understanding Hair PH, hair is best healthy when kept in the PH range of 4.5 to 5.5 and relaxers have a PH range of 11-14! This is highly corrosive but is used to caused permanent "controlled damage" to your hair and because of this, you should wait until your hair is a desired state of health before using relaxers again!

9 THINNING WITH AGE

Many of us wish that we could never age or feel the weight of aging on our bodies and minds but unfortunately, we will all age with every passing year. When you are young and energetic, your body has the ability to handle infections, viruses, diseases and injuries phenomenally better than your body can in old age. The benefit also to being younger is a higher metabolism that helps to maintain a more fit body, tighter more youthful skin, and a head full of hair!

Many women and men who age notice that their hair becomes thinner as time passes and this is most noticeable to those who remembered having a thick head full of hair in their younger days! The reason why many at an older age begin to have thinning hair is because your hormonal balance changes within your body. As you age, your hormones aren't raging as much as they used to in your young days and because of this, estrogen levels will begin to decrease after a certain age , usually starting in your late 20's to mid 30's. As estrogen levels within the body decrease overtime, in both men and women, this leads to a production of DHT. As you age, its effects are what we visually see as pattern baldness.

DHT (Dihydrotestosterone): an enzyme that develops with the conversion of testosterone and Type II 5-alpha reductase, which is located in the oil gland of your hair follicle

Pattern baldness is a normal encounter many will or can endure in their lifetime. If Thickening Hair Oils still do not help you in reversing your thin hair, and even a change in diet doesn't help (Dieting For Hair Growth Manual), surgical hair restoration is also an option!

10 SURGICAL HAIR RESTORATION

Surgical hair restoration is only suggested for those who have truly given every home made remedy and diet plan a fair and independent chance. Before going under the knife, give each individual Thickening Hair Oil Recipe and a diet rich in specific vitamins and nutrients its chance to produce results within a time frame of 2 to 4 months.

Taking a natural approach to growing back thin or thinning hair is at a lower price point than surgery offers but it is still completely up to you and understandable to seek surgical hair restoration and there are two options you can take to surgically restore your thin hair permanently!

FUE Hair Transplant: Follicular Unit Extraction
FUT Hair Transplant: Follicular Unit Transplant

The FUE transplant requires individual follicles to be extracted from your scalp after injecting a local anesthesia to the preferred area of extraction. This procedure involves implanting individual follicles throughout your thinning or bald area of scalp. A positive to this procedure is that it does not require staples/stiches, leaves behind no scars and requires little recovery time. The negative is that it can take multiple procedures to achieve your desired result of density.

The FUT transplant requires a thin patch of scalp removed preferably from the back of your head after injecting a local anesthesia. This procedure involves dissecting your scalp into patches of 2 to 4 follicle units that will be inserted into your desired scalp area. The positive of this procedure is that it can be done in one session. The negative is that it can leave behind a scar, requires staples/stiches and has a lengthy recovery time.

AFTERWORDS

"This manual was made in mind for those who desire step by step help with growing back their thinning hair in a way that allows you to try a variety of solutions. As you may have read throughout these chapters, this manual is condensed with a wide variety of solutions for achieving healthy thicker hair whether you decide to go the natural or surgical route. You may have chosen to read this guide because you support my work, you were looking for information on growing thicker hair, or you were looking for this information to help a loved one.

Personally, I have never had problems with thin or thinning hair considering the fact that the edges of my hair is thinner in comparison to the rest of my hair. The edges of my hair and the nape are a little bit finer and at a lower density than the rest of my hair. This does not bother me and I have never had problems with breakage or thinning on my edges because I take great care of my hair and something that has been golden for retaining length on my edge hairs, has been from two strand twisting medium to small sections of just my edge hairs to limit the amount of manipulation it encounters. I constantly receive an overwhelming amount of emails daily from women and men, who need help with their hair and the majority of these emails, consist of help with growing back the edges of their hair or to reverse thinning. This manual is inspired by those who need my help in this way! Reversing your thin hair is possible!

I hope that you thoroughly enjoyed this read, it was a pleasure of mine to write this for your knowledge and enjoyment."

Sincerely, Breanna

ADDITIONAL RESOURCES

The Official Website: www.Howtoblackhair.com

The Online Store: www.HowtoblackhairStore.com

Free Subscription Email: http://eepurl.com/FZs5b

For Additional Hair Questions

YourHairQuestions@Gmail.com

Black Hair Styling Tutorials

BlackWomenHair YouTube Channel

www.Youtube.com/BlackWomenHair

HowToBlackHair YouTube Channel

www.Youtube.com/HowToBlackHair

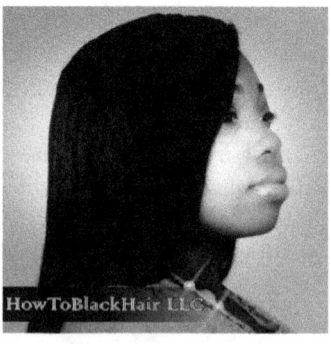

The Natural Hair Bible

The 10 Commandments of Black Hair Care

www.HowToBlackHair.com

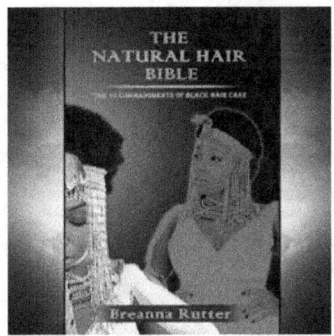

The Relaxed Hair Bible

The 10 Commandments of Long Healthy Relaxed Hair

www.HowToBlackHair.com

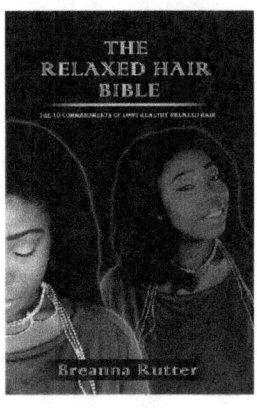

Black Hair Styling DVDs (Over 20+ Hairstyles)

www.HowToBlackHair.com

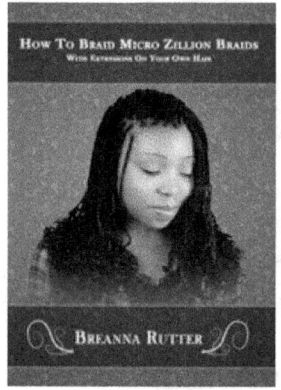 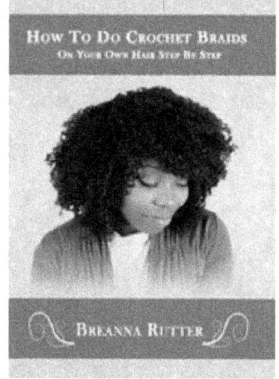

DEFINITION GUIDE

Course Hair: *your individual strands of hair are the same size or bigger in size (diameter) to regular sewing thread*

Cuticles: *a naturally protecting shield (arranged like shingles to the roof of a home) outside of your hair strands*

Dermal Papilla: *a raised dermis located underneath the root of your follicle that houses the blood supply*

DHT (Dihydrotestosterone): *an enzyme that develops with the conversion of testosterone and Type II 5-alpha reductase, which is located in the oil gland of your hair follicle*

Follicle: *an individual strand of hair*

FUE Hair Transplant: *Follicular Unit Extraction*

FUT Hair Transplant: *Follicular Unit Transplant*

Thick Hair: *your ponytail width, with all of your hair gathered, is the width of a quarter or larger*

Thin Hair: *your ponytail width, with all of your hair gathered, is the width of a nickel or smaller*

INDEX

HOW TO BLACK HAIR LLC.
WRITTEN BY BREANNA RUTTER
BOOK DESIGNED BY BREANNA RUTTER
COVER DESIGNED BY JARED RUTTER
ALL RIGHTS RESERVED.
VISIT WWW.HOWTOBLACKHAIR.COM

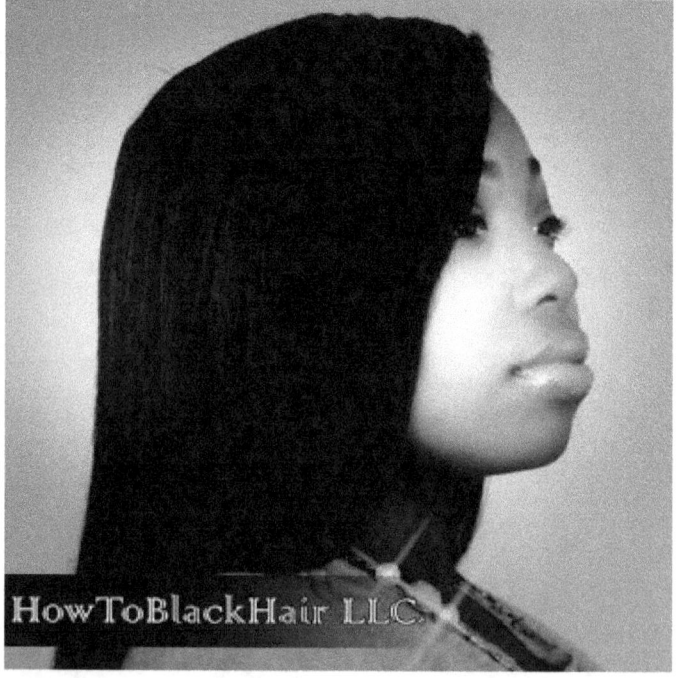